MW01600894

HOW TO NATURALLY REMOVE CANCER FROM THE BODY

This book is not intended as a substitute for medical advice from a qualified physician. The intent of this book is to provide accurate general information in regard to the subject matter covered. If medical advice or other expert help is needed, the services of an appropriate medical professional should be sought.

Table of Contents

Preface

Humanity, especially those among us entrapped in the concrete jungles of the earth have not only lost sight of true health, but also of the life force that permeates all things. The paradise that is our Earth, the flowers, the trees, the flowing waters, the animals, that what gives us life and true joy has been lost. Because of this, we are now being controlled by a pharmaceutical industry that only perceives us as a means to maximize profits.

The pharmaceutical industry controls the medical curriculum of universities. By design, none of the aspiring medical professionals are instructed in human nutrition. Unless someone is a specialist the only thing the pediatrician is taught to do is look at your symptoms and prescribe a pharmaceutical drug.

But not only that, the pharmaceutical industry controls all the major "medical" research. The research that they sponsor is designed to sabotage potential natural cures and to promulgate addictive drugs that address symptoms.

If someone desires to find a cure for a particular disease, there are thousands of research articles(located in databases like Pubmed) authored by International scientists and universities that are beyond the tentacles of the pharmaceutical industry.

But unfortunately, most people are conditioned not to read or research, much less take responsibility and control of their own health. The masses have been conditioned to blindly listen and obey.

Introduction

What is Cancer

Cancer is a group of more than 100 different diseases. It can develop almost anywhere in the body. Cells are the basic units that make up the human body. Cells grow and divide to make new cells as the body needs them. Typically, when cells die due to age or damage, new cells replace them. Cancer takes root when "genetic" changes interfere with this orderly process. Cells then start to grow uncontrollably forming tumors, which can be cancerous or benign. A cancerous tumor can grow and proliferate to other parts of the body, while benign tumor means can grow but will not spread.

Some cancers do not form a tumors. These include leukemias, a majority of lymphomas, and myeloma.

Types of cancer

Cancer is categorized based on its genesis within the body. The four main types of cancer are:

- **Carcinomas.** A carcinoma begins in the skin or the tissue that covers the surface of internal organs and glands. They are the most common

- type of cancer. Examples include **prostate cancer**, **breast cancer**, **lung cancer**, and **colorectal cancer**.
- **Sarcomas.** A **sarcoma** takes root in connective tissue. It can develop in fat, muscles, nerves, tendons, joints, blood vessels, lymph vessels, cartilage, or bone.
- **Leukemias.** Leukemia develops in the blood, healthy blood cells change and begin to grow uncontrollably. The 4 main types of leukemia are **acute lymphocytic leukemia**, **chronic lymphocytic leukemia**, **acute myeloid leukemia**, and **chronic myeloid leukemia**.
- **Lymphomas.** Lymphoma spreads within the lymphatic system. The lymphatic system is a network of vessels and glands that help fight infection. There are 2 main
- types of lymphomas: **Hodgkin lymphoma** and **non-Hodgkin lymphoma**

How cancer spreads

When a cancerous tumor grows, the bloodstream or lymphatic system can transport the cancer cells to other parts of the body. During this process known as metastasis, the cancer cells grow and may develop into new tumors.

Cancer often spreads is to the lymph nodes. Lymph nodes are tiny, bean-shaped organs that help fight infection. They are located in clusters in different parts of the body, such as the neck, groin area, and under the arms.

Cancer may also spread through the bloodstream to distant parts of the body, such as the bones, liver, lungs, or brain. Even in cancer mestasisis, it's still categorized based on the area of its origin. For example, if breast cancer spreads to the lungs, it is metastatic breast cancer, not lung cancer.

Chapter 1

What is the cause of Cancer?

Cancer is caused by all the carcinogenic poisons we allow into our body, by way of food source(herbicides, pesticides,GMOs), inhalation(pollution, smoking), and the skin(materials, chemicals). Being that modern humans in western societies are all malnourished of minerals, whole complex food derived vitamins, and antioxidants. This allows cancer to easily take root within the human body.

As you can see from this map statistically, America and western Europe have the highest incidents of all cancers.

It's almost impossible to live in America not to know someone who has or knows someone battling cancer.

Genetically engineered organisms(GMOS)

If you consume processed food, it's near impossible not to be ingesting GMOs unless the product says organic, but in America organic does not mean 100% organic.

On the USDA Organic website it states:

"Organic"

- Any product that contains a minimum of 95 percent organic ingredients (excluding salt and water)
- Up to 5 percent of ingredients may be nonorganic agricultural products and/or nonagricultural products on the <u>National List</u> (nonorganic agricultural products and several nonagricultural products on the National List may only be used if they are not commercially available as organic)

So even with "organic", you're still possibly getting GMO's and synthetic pesticides. The GMO industry is very strong and controls the FDA and much of the so-called research on the safety of ingesting genetically engineered foods. Any research that has been revealed the GMO industry tries to discredit it in every possible way.

There was a study posted in 2012 by researchers led by Gilles-Eric Séralini at the University of Caen in France announced evidence for a raft of health problems in rats fed maize that has been modified to be resistant to the herbicide Roundup. They also found similar health problems in rats fed the herbicide itself.

The rodents experienced hormone imbalances and more and bigger breast tumours, earlier in life, than rats fed a non-GM diet, the researchers claim. The GM- or pesticide-fed rats also died earlier.

In my view, avoid GMOs like the plague, eat what nature designed for you to eat, not what was created in some corporations secretive laboratory.

Carcinogenic Pesticides & Herbicides

Pesticides are chemicals used to get rid of undesired plants or organism that may hinder the growth of the main plantation. These can be rodents, water plants, bugs, and many more. The production of pesticide helps to ensure the product of plantation will grow vast and with flawless result. Early pesticide used organic and natural compound. However, as technology advanced, pesticides are made from synthetic chemicals and not all of them are safe. There may be some that are carcinogenic.

Studies have linked synthetic pesticides to a variety of chronic health conditions such as diabetes, cancer, and neurological defects. Carbamates and organophosphates are known to affect the nervous system by disrupting a neurotransmitter called acetylcholine. Studies have shown preliminary evidence that chronic, low-dose exposure to pesticides increases the risk of cognitive impairments and diseases such as Alzheimer's and Parkinson's disease. A study of 50 pesticides and more than 30,000 licensed pesticide applicators linked exposure of seven pesticides that contain chlorinated compounds (including two herbicides, two organophosphate insecticides, and two organochlorines) to increased risk of diabetes. Exposure to pesticides has also been associated with increased infertility in women and developmental problems in children.

The March/April 2013 issue of *CA: A Cancer Journal for Clinicians* published a review by the U.S. National Cancer Institute reporting the widespread recognition that exposure (through food, water, skin and air) to many different pesticides are convincingly linked to an increase in cancer risk.

This is an important acknowledgement, as this appears in one of the most widely read medical journals published by the American Cancer Society.

The authors present a clear picture of the link between pesticide exposure and the following cancer types:

- Breast cancer
- Prostate cancer
- Leukemia
- Lymphoma
- Multiple myeloma
- although these cancers are the most recognized for their association with pesticide exposure, many others have been linked in studies (i.e. lung, pancreatic, brain, stomach, ovarian, kidney, etc.)

Glyphosate, an herbicide that remains the world's most popular weed killer, raises the cancer risk of those exposed to it by 41%, a new analysis says. Researchers from the University of Washington evaluated existing studies into the chemical glyphosate, found in weed killers including Monsanto's popular Roundup, and concluded that it significantly increases the risk of non-Hodgkin lymphoma, a cancer of the immune system.

Carcinogenics in Cosmetics

The laws governing cosmetics and personal care products are so limited that known cancer-causing chemicals(carcinogens) are legally allowed in personal care products. Some carcinogens, such as formaldehyde and formaldehyde releasing preservatives, are common in personal care products, while others are less common, but still occasionally present.

Formaldehyde

Formaldehyde is intentionally added to some products, such as keratin hair straighteners. Formaldehyde-releasing preservatives (FRPs) are also widely used in personal care products including nail polish, eye shadow, mascara, nail treatment, shampoo and blush for the prevention of bacterial growth. FRPs are designed to release formaldehyde slowly and constantly over time to act as a preservative.

IARC, the National Toxicology Program (NTP) and California EPA's Proposition 65 (Prop 65) classify formaldehyde as a human carcinogen. EPA identifies formaldehyde as a probable human carcinogen. The National Institute of Occupational Safety and Health (NIOSH) also raises concern that exposure to formaldehyde leads to irritation of the eyes, nose, throat and respiratory system.Standards for cosmetics in Japan prohibit formaldehyde use in cosmetics, and the European Commission restricts formaldehyde in cosmetics to no more than five percent concentration in the finished product.

Phenacetin

Phenacetin was used as pain and fever reducer until banned in the US by the Food and Drug Administration in 1983 due to its carcinogenicity.

Although it is no longer used as a drug, it is still occasionally used in personal care products as a stabilizer in products such as facial hair bleach, hair color and women's depilatories.

Prop 65 identify phenacetin as a human carcinogen. Phenacetin can also cause renal damage and anemia. Exposure to phenacetin has been linked malignant mammary tumors.

Coal Tar

Coal tar is a known carcinogen and a by-product from coal processing. It is used in cosmetics containing hair dyes, shampoos, dandruff/scalp treatment and redness/rosacea treatment.

IARC, NTP and EPA classify coal tar as a known human carcinogen. Coal tar was one of the first occupational exposures linked to cancer; when scrotal cancer among young chimney sweeps was associated with exposure. It is also associated with cancers of the lung, bladder, kidney, and digestive tract. Environmental Canada classifies that coal tar pitch is persistent and inherently toxic to aquatic organisms. European Commission prohibits coal tar use in cosmetics.

Coal tars are complex mixtures that can contain other known carcinogens, such as polycyclic aromatic hydrocarbons (PAHs), such as benzoapyrene. PAHs damage DNA, and exposure to PAHs can lead to tumors on lungs, bladder and skin; and PAHs can also cause non-cancer toxicities like reproductive and developmental toxicity.

Benzene

Benzene is derived from coal tar, and exposure routes of benzene are inhalation and ingestion. Benzene is used in the production of plastics and detergents and occasionally in hair conditioner and styling lotion. IARC and NTP classify benzene as a known human carcinogen. Prop 65 identifies benzene as a concern for both cancer and developmental toxicity, and benzene can lead to mammary tumors in female mice. EPA identifies benzene as a known human respiratory toxicant. Benzene is considered a priority pollutant of wastewater by EPA, which means environmental releases of benzene are regulated. The Endocrine Disruption Exchange considers benzene as an endocrine disruptor. Occupational exposure to benzene is linked to leukemia; and benzene can target organs including eyes, skin, respiratory system, blood, central nervous system and bone marrow. The European Commission prohibits benzene use in cosmetics, and it is restricted in the Convention for the Protection of the Marine Environment of the North-East Atlantic (OSPAR).

Mineral oils (untreated and mildly treated)

Mineral oils are derived from crude oil, and mildly refined mineral oils always contain significant amounts of PAHs. Mineral oils are common in a wide array of personal care products, including eye shadow, moisturizer, lip gloss, lipstick, conditioner, hair color and bleaching, facial treatment, styling gel/lotion, blush and concealer. IARC, NTP and Prop 65 classify untreated and mildly treated mineral oils as a known human carcinogen. NIOSH raises concerns that mineral oils can target organs including eyes, skin, and respiratory system though inhalation, or skin and eye contact.

Ethylene oxide

Ethylene oxide is a possible impurity in personal care products as a byproduct of the process of ethoxylation, which is used to buffer the harsh effects of some sudsing agents; Ethylene oxide is most widely used to sterilize medical instruments.

It can be found in tobacco smoke, automobile exhausts, and foods. There is strong evidence that ethylene oxide can lead lymphatic and hematopoietic cancers; and some studies found increased incidence of breast cancer in exposed workers. Prop 65 identifies ethylene oxide as a concern for both cancer and developmental toxicity in both females and males. The Endocrine Disruption Exchange lists ethylene oxide as an endocrine disruptor. NIOSH concludes that ethylene oxide leads peritoneal cancer and leukemia; exposure to ethylene oxide through inhalation, ingestion, and skin and eye contact can disrupt respiratory system, central nervous system, and reproductive system.The European Commission prohibits ethylene oxide use in cosmetics.

Heavy Metals

Heavy metals like hexavalent chromium, and cadmium serve as colorants in eye shadow and lip gloss. Other metals such as arsenic are impurities in cosmetic ingredients including facial lotion, shampoo, and foundation as a result of arsenic contamination in ingredients such as D&C Red 6, aluminum starch octenylsuccinate, hydrogenated cottonseed oil, and polyvinyl acetate.

IARC, the National Toxicology Program and California's Prop 65 identify cadmium and its compounds, arsenic, and chromium as human carcinogens; in addition, chromium can also lead to developmental problems in both females and males.

Cadmium and its compounds

In addition to its carcinogenic properties, cadmium targets the cardiovascular, renal, neurological, reproductive and respiratory systems through inhalation and ingestion.

Standards for cosmetics in Japan and European Commission prohibit use of cadmium compounds in cosmetics.

Arsenic

The U.S. Environmental Protection Agency (EPA) concludes that there is sufficient evidence that arsenic is a carcinogen; and arsenic can also lead hyperpigmentation, keratosis and possible vascular complications. EPA lists arsenic as a priority pollutant and regulates arsenic emissions; The Endocrine Disruption Exchange suggests that arsenic can cause endocrine disruption. NIOSH demonstrates that exposure to arsenic leads to lung and lymphatic cancer; because it can target organs including liver, kidneys, skin, lungs and lymphatic system through inhalation, skin absorption, skin and eye contact, and ingestion.

The European Commission prohibits arsenic in cosmetics.

Chromium

The European Chemicals Agency (ECHA) lists chromium as a carcinogen and mutagen. NIOSH indicates that exposure to chromium leads to lung cancer; and the metal targets organs including blood, respiratory system, liver and kidneys. It can cause increased blood leukocytes, eye injury, and skin ulcers through inhalation, ingestion, and skin and eye contact. EPA considers chromium to be both bioaccumulative and ecotoxic. The European Commission prohibits chromium use in cosmetics.

Silica

Silica occurs in two different forms: **crystalline** or **amorphous**; quartz is the common mineral in crystalline silica. Respirable crystalline silica is an airborne contaminant that can penetrate the lung when it is inhaled.

Crystalline silica is widely used in lipsticks, lip gloss, eye shadow, eye liner, foundation, sunscreen, lotion and shampoo.

NTP and IARC both list crystalline silica of respirable size as a known human carcinogen, and Prop 65 classifies silica, crystalline (airborne particles of respirable size) as a carcinogen. NIOSH raises concerns about lung cancer in animals exposed to crystalline silica; and this chemical can target eyes and the respiratory system through inhalation, and skin and eye contact.

How to Avoid These Chemicals?

Read labels and avoid cosmetics and personal care products containing formaldehyde and formaldehyde-releasing preservatives (quaternium-15, diazolidinyl urea, imidazolidinyl urea, DMDM hydantoin, and 2-bromo-2-nitropropane-1,3 diol), phenacetin, coal tar, benzene, untreated or mildly treated mineral oils, ethylene oxide, chromium, cadmium and its compounds, arsenic and crystalline silica (or quartz).

Carcinogens in Cleaning Products

As more accurate methods for diagnosing cancers become standard practice, greater emphasis is put on eliminating preventable cancers. The air in our homes is filled with potentially carcinogenic compounds released by: Air fresheners, Detergents, Fabric softeners, Disinfectants, and Deodorants.

The lifetime risk of cancer from air pollutants, including those from indoor cleaning products, is estimated to be 0.06 to 0.1 (or 60 to 100 people for every 1,000).

A study published in 2010 identified that women who extensively used cleaning products, were twice as likely to have been diagnosed with breast cancer. This article reviews the most common ingredients in cleaning products, and the evidence for their ability to cause cancer.

How Are Cancer Causing Ingredients Classified?

It can be difficult to determine the cancer risk of an ingredient, with the FDA and EU frequently coming to different conclusions. Both regulatory bodies review reports published by the World

Health Organization's (WHO) independent 'International Agency for Research on Cancer' (IARC), which classifies compounds into five categories of carcinogenicity.

Classification	Definition
Group 1	Carcinogenic to humans
Group 2A	Probably carcinogenic to humans
Group 2B	Possibly carcinogenic to humans
Group 3	Not classifiable as carcinogenic to humans
Group 4	Probably not carcinogenic to humans

1. Phthalates (e.g. dibutylphthalate, diethylphthalate)

Used for: A plasticizer used to soften plastics, stabilize fragrances, and found in many aerosol air fresheners. Phthalates are not chemically bound to plastics, and so can leech from plastic packaging.

WHO Classification: 2B (possibly carcinogenic to humans)

Evidence: Many everyday items contain phthalates, with low levels present in children's toys, infant formula, and the enteric coatings of medications; phthalates can be detected in the urine of most adults. A 2010 study showed significantly higher levels of urinary phthalates in women with breast cancer. In laboratory studies, phthalates have been shown to imitate estrogen ('xenoestrogens') and generate genomic instability, which may explain the increased breast tumor growth seen in laboratory studies

2. Chlorinated Bleaches (e.g. sodium hypochlorite)

Used for: Household bleaches are used in cleaning products to disinfect, remove stains, and deodorize.

WHO Classification: 3 (not classifiable as to its carcinogenicity to humans)

Ingredient Labels: 'Bleach', 'bleaching agents', 'chlorine-based bleach'

Evidence: There no evidence to suggest that chlorinated bleaches are directly carcinogenic, although regular inhalation has been associated with fatal chronic obstructive pulmonary disease. There is concern that chlorinated byproducts (trichloromethane and tetrachloromethane) may be released into the air when using bleach. These can cause liver, kidney, and bladder cancers, but at concentrations higher than would expected to be released by bleach (e.g. contaminated drinking water).

3. Parabens (e.g. methylparaben, ethylparaben)

Used for: Used as preservatives in a wide range of household products, parabens inhibit the growth of bacteria and fungus, prolonging shelf-lives.

WHO Classification: Not listed

Ingredient Labels: 'Preservatives', or those ending in '-paraben' ('methylparaben')

Evidence: Like phthalates, parabens have been shown to be xenoestrogens, and are detectable in many urine samples. Since the 1990s, evidence has suggested that parabens can stimulate growth of breast cancer cells, and in 2004 unmetabolized parabens were identified in human breast cancer samples for the first time. A 2011 study correlated paraben concentration to damaged sperm DNA. Parabens are known to stimulate cancer cells at high doses in the short-term, but it's still not clear if low-dose accumulation can cause cancer in humans.

4. Quaternary Ammonium Compounds (e.g. benzalkonium chloride, tetraethylammonium bromide)

Used for: Cationic surfactants used to reduce surface tension, dispersing dirt, increasing the effectiveness of detergents and fabric softeners. Commonly used as preservatives.

WHO Classification: Not listed

Ingredient Labels: 'Preservatives', 'benzalkonium chloride', 'quaternium-15'

Evidence: Quaternary ammonium compounds are widely used as preservatives in pharmaceutical eye drops and nasal sprays, and at higher concentrations in shampoos. The evidence for carcinogenicity is controversial, and currently lab-based. In 2006 a study showed DNA damage in exposed lung tissue, backed by a 2007 study showing DNA damage in liver and white blood cells. In contrast, a 2005 study found no evidence of cancer activity in mammalian cells.

5. Linear Alkylbenzene Sulfonates (LAS)

Used for: Anionic surfactants used to reduce surface tension, dispersing dirt, increasing the effectiveness of cleaning products. Commonly found in laundry detergents.

WHO Classification: Not listed

Ingredient Labels: 'Anionic surfactants', 'linear alkylbenzenesulfonates', 'LAS'

Evidence: Since the late 1980s, concern has been raised on the accumulation of linear alkylbenzene sulfonates (LAS) in the environment. In treated sewage, LAS concentrations are found between

0.008 – 6mg/mL. LAS is considered non-toxic and non-carcinogenic to aquatic organisms. A 2016 study highlighted the lack of human data and found that at very low concentrations (1-15parts per million) LAS increased the growth rate of colon tumor cells in the laboratory.

6. Phenols (e.g. 2-phenylphenol (OPP))

Used for: Phenols are used in low concentrations as preservatives in many household products, and in higher concentrations as disinfectants (hospitals use phenolic disinfectants to sterilize medical equipment).

WHO Classification: 3 (not classifiable as to its carcinogenicity to humans)

Ingredient Labels: 'Preservatives', 'phenols', 'o-phenylphenol', 'phenylphenate'

Evidence: The evidence for 2-phenylphenol (OPP) carcinogenicity is of generally low quality, especially in humans. Rats fed 0.5% to 4% OPP in the diets over 13 weeks developed the early signs of bladder tumors, a result replicated in other rat studies – but notably, not in other species. In two humans fatally exposed to 10grams of OPP, toxic effects were noted on bladder linings. In contrast, OPP is rapidly excreted from the human body, and so the accumulation of low doses is unlikely, even on repeated exposure.

7. Triclosan (TCS)

Used for: A preservative used to prolong the shelf-lives of detergents, by inhibiting the growth of bacteria and fungus. The effectiveness of triclosan has been questioned by the FDA, with a risk of promoting bacterial resistance without inhibiting growth.

WHO Classification: Not listed

Ingredient Labels: 'Preservatives', 'triclosan', 'TCS'

Evidence: The widespread use of triclosan in household and personal care products make it one of the most common pollutants worldwide, detectable in aquatic life and human breastmilk. The compound is estrogenic and androgenic, and so may disrupt hormone regulation, but baboons given 300mg/kg/day for a year in 1975 experienced no carcinogenic or other abnormal effects (other than intermittent diarrhea). A 2010 review concluded that triclosan is not carcinogenic to humans.

8. Ethanolamines (e.g. diethanolamine (DEA), triethanolamine (TEA))

Used for: Commonly used as emulsifiers to bind water-soluble and fatty ingredients in cleaning products like laundry detergents, washing liquids, and hand sanitizers.**WHO Classification:** Diethanolamine 2B (possibly carcinogenic to humans); triethanolamine 3 (not classifiable as to its carcinogenicity to humans)

Ingredient Labels: 'Nonionic surfactants', 'diethanolamine', 'DEA', 'triethanolamine', 'TEA'

Evidence: The carcinogenicity of the ethanolamines is thought to be due to their structural similarity to choline, an essential nutrient produced in the liver. In animal studies, there is evidence for this link, and long-term accumulation of low-dose diethanolamine has been shown to cause the formation of liver and kidney tumors. Choline is essential for neuronal development, and in mice, diethanolamine accelerates cell death in fetal neurons. There is very little evidence for the carcinogenic effects of ethanolamines in humans, and the WHO classification is based on animal studies.

10. 1,4-Dioxane

Used for: A volatile organic compound (VOC), 1,4-dioxane is used as a solvent in the manufacture of many ingredients in cleaning products. The compound is not specifically added by manufacturers but may be present as a contaminant.

WHO Classification: 2B (possibly carcinogenic to humans)
Ingredient Labels: As a contaminant will not be listed on ingredient labels

Evidence: 1,4-dioxane concentrations in personal care and cleaning products are becoming increasingly concerning because the compound is rated as possibly carcinogenic by both WHO and US EPA. These classifications are from animal data concluding exposure significantly increases the risk of liver, gallbladder, and nasal cancer. Three small human studies (less than 200 people) published in the 1970s evaluating historic 1,4-dioxane exposure found no increased cancer risk. Manufacturers are not legally required to remove 1,4-dioxane, although the FDA monitors levels.

11. Polychlorinated Biphenyls (Endocrine Disruptor)

Used for: Not directly added to detergents, but there is a risk that polychlorinated biphenyls may be produced as a byproduct of the manufacturing of detergent ingredients.

WHO Classification: 1 (carcinogenic to humans)

Ingredient Labels: As a possible contaminant will not be listed on ingredient labels

Evidence: The use and production of polychlorinated biphenyls has been banned in most countries since the early 1980s due to their direct genotoxic and mutagenic activity, known as 'dioxin-like'. Large population studies repeatedly identified polychlorinated biphenyls as an occupational exposure correlated with diagnoses of melanoma, breast cancer, and non-Hodgkin lymphoma. In addition, the compounds are known to alter thyroid function and have estrogenic activity (endocrine disruptors).

How Real Are the Risks?

It can be difficult to establish how likely a compound is to cause cancer. Without human trials, the risk is extrapolated from lab results, theoretical mechanisms, and retrospective epidemiological studies. For the compounds listed above, a WHO classification of 1, 2A, or 2B are a reasonable cancer risk in sufficient concentrations, and exposure should be reduced if possible.

Are There Alternatives?

If using commercial cleaning products, the best way to avoid the most harmful ingredients is to check the product is 'free' of the ingredient (e.g. 'phthalate-free' will normally be prominently displayed). This is more difficult for compounds used in manufacturing, such as crystalline silica. For these, the only way to avoid exposure is to use cleaning products with fewer, safer ingredients.

A simpler cleaning product is baking soda and vinegar, with warm water. This has the advantage of avoiding potentially carcinogenic ingredients, but it can be difficult to remove tougher stains. There are several 'natural' cleaning products that only contain a few ingredients, but these are generally more expensive, and care needs to be taken to ensure the ingredients are safer.

Most people will find it difficult to eliminate all commercial cleaning products from their day-to-day lives, my advise is to use only use plant based bio-degrable products. But some practical steps to reduce carcinogen exposure include:

- Only use cleaning products in well-ventilated areas
- Stand the recommended distance away when using cleaning products
- Use the smallest quantities possible, and only for difficult to remove stains
- Avoid using aerosol products that pollute the air (e.g. air fresheners)

Carcinogens in Plastics

On Jan. 27, 2020 the Environmental Defense Fund, along with several other organizations, submitted a petition to the Food and Drug Administration that urged the agency to limit the use of the chemical bisphenol-A (BPA) in food packaging. BPA is just one of many chemicals used in plastics that are concerning because of their links to certain health conditions.

While I supports stricter limits on the use of BPA, the F.D.A. is "grossly outdated" in its approach to regulating chemicals used in food packaging. Focusing on a single chemical like BPA rather than the entire suite of harmful chemicals in plastics and other materials leads to chemicals geting replaced with something very similar or that may be equally as problematic.

Given this reality, here's what you need to know about how chemicals in plastics and other consumer products might affect your health and how you can lower your exposure.

Plastics may look inert, but the chemicals inside them are not. There are chemicals used in plastics that are not tightly bound to the material, which means they easily leach away, especially when exposed to heat.

The two most concerning types of chemicals in plastics are **phthalates** and **bisphenols**. Phthalates, which are typically added to plastics to make them pliable and soft, are used in plastic food wrap, vinyl flooring and personal care products ,such as, deodorants, nail polish, hair gels, shampoos, soaps and lotions. Bisphenols, including BPA, are more typically found in hard polycarbonate plastics such as water and juice bottles, food containers, eyeglass lenses and have been identified in the linings of food and soda cans.

In the research article "The Endocrine Society's Second Scientific Statement on Endocrine-Disrupting Chemicals", suggests that phthalates and bisphenols can act as endocrine disruptors, meaning that they either mimic or interfere with hormones in the body. The early troubling studies of phthalates and bisphenols were on rodents, but more recently, researchers have begun linking the chemicals to worrying effects on humans, Dr. Trasande said.

For example, human studies have found that exposure to higher phthalate levels in the womb is associated with asthma in childhood. And in boys, it's linked to more behavioral problems and shorter distances between their anuses and genitals — a measure linked to lower testosterone levels and semen quality later in life. In men, higher phthalate exposures in adulthood have been associated with lowered sperm counts; and exposures in pregnant women have been linked to lower thyroid hormone levels and more preterm births.

BPA, on the other hand, can mimic estrogen, another hormone important to reproductive development and function, and has been linked to reduced fertility in men and women, later puberty in girls, earlier puberty in boys and behavioral problems in children.

There's also growing evidence that exposure to hormone disruptors like phthalates and bisphenols is associated with a greater risk of Type 2 diabetes, heart disease and obesity. In a 2021 review, researchers noted that exposure to these and other endocrine disruptors from food, consumer products and the environment may increase the risk of obesity by a similar magnitude as more commonly cited culprits like lack of exercise or following a poor diet.

The good news is that phthalates and bisphenols don't stay in your body permanently, so making changes has a near-immediate effect. If you reduce your exposure, you can wash out these chemicals from your body within a matter of days.

Prioritize fresh, whole foods.

Studies have shown that people who consume more fresh foods and fewer processed and packaged foods have lower urinary concentrations of BPA and phthalates.

Processed meals, like those purchased from fast food restaurants or grocery stores (think boxed macaroni and cheese) can be convenient and sometimes necessary, but they can contain high levels of phthalates. Studies also suggest that higher-fat foods, like certain meat and dairy products, can accumulate more phthalates than others. Bisphenols and other chemicals can lurk in the linings of cans, so soups, sauces and beverages packaged in glass tend to be safer choice, as are fresh or frozen fruits and veggies. The plastic bags used for frozen produce don't contain phthalates or bisphenols, and cold temperatures make leaching of chemicals from plastic much less likely.

Avoid using certain types of plastic containers.

Bisphenols can hide in the plastics used to store food and drinks, so when possible, use metal or glass versions of baby bottles, sippy cups, food storage containers and water bottles. The F.D.A. banned BPA from baby bottles and sippy cups in 2012 and in infant formula packaging in 2013, but products labeled "BPA-free" might be made with other bisphenols with similar health effects.

When you use plastic, look at the recycling code on the bottom for clues about what's in it. Dr. Trasande recommended avoiding items labeled 3 for phthalates, 7 for bisphenols and 6 for styrene. (Styrene, which is found in Styrofoam and other plastic products, is a human carcinogen, according to the National Institutes of Health.) also avoid plastic wrap and dispose of plastics that are scratched or that are showing signs of wear.

Avoid heating plastics.

Warming plastics by heating them in the microwave, using them for hot foods or washing them in the dishwasher can increase the chance that harmful chemicals will leach from them and end up in your food or liquid. Swap out vinyl products. If you have a vinyl shower curtain, switching to one made with fabric is an easy way to reduce phthalates in your home. Also watch out for vinyl in products like anti-slip bathtub mats, baby play mats and place mats, and choose products made from other materials.

Reduce exposures from toys.

Phthalates used to be in soft plastic toys, but they were banned in 2008 from toys in the United States. Still, if your baby is in a stage from 6 months to a year when they want to put everything in their mouth, try to direct them toward wooden or silicone toys instead, Dr. Sathyanarayana said. Simply playing with plastic toys is fine, she added.

Take care with personal care products.

Cosmetics, nail polish, shampoo, body wash, lotions and powders often contain phthalates, and use of these products may explain why women have higher phthalate levels in their bodies than men. Recent research has also found that Black and Hispanic women in the United States have greater phthalate exposure, including during pregnancy.

Choosing personal care products labeled "phthalate-free" or "fragrance-free" (phthalates are often found in fragrances) can significantly reduce phthalate exposure.

Reduce exposure to dust.

Phthalates can be found in glues, adhesives (such as those found on tape), carpet backings, vinyl shower curtains and floors, and other soft pliable plastics. These chemicals can wind up in the dust in your home, and then enter the body by inhalation or absorption through the skin, or hand-to-mouth activity of babies and young children. I recommend using a vacuum cleaner outfitted with a HEPA filter. Without the filter, the vacuum just blows the fine phthalate particles out the back end, he explained.

Chapter 2

What is the anti-cancer diet?

The anti-cancer diet is a cancer preventative diet, and it has three components consisting of naturally occurring alkaline water, nutrition, and antioxidants.

Alkaline Water

Drinking natural alkaline daily, not ionized water, is very important is preventing the development of cancer. The chemical makeup of natural alkaline water is significantly different from ionized water. Water ionizers split apart water molecules with electricity to artificially create a high pH value. While natural alkaline water has a high pH value because of the presence of key minerals the body needs to function properly, such as calcium, potassium, sodium, and magnesium.

What makes alkaline water essential in the prevention of cancer is its ability to neutralize acids. Body acidity accelerates free radical damage and premature aging. Acidosis leads to partial lipid breakdown and destructive oxidative cascades, accelerating free radical damage of cell walls and intracellular membrane structures. In the process, many healthy cells are destroyed. It has been proven in the research article "Oxidative stress, inflammation, and cancer: How are they linked? ", that cancer initiation and progression has been linked to oxidative stress by increasing DNA mutations or inducing DNA damage, genome instability, and cell proliferation.

Nutrition

Getting correct nutrition is the basis of all health, not just for preventing the development of cancer.

Getting proper nutrition from our foods, if we live in America is near impossible. Due to the fact that the commercial farm soils have been depleted of minerals decades ago from over farming. The majority of commercial fertilizers used for foods crops only contain nitrogen, phosphorus, and potassium, which is only three of the major and trace minerals that are essential for human life.

That being said we want to procure organic wholefoods that we can cook, we need to avoid processed foods and as much as possible, even if they are labelled organic. Processed foods have little nutritional value. We also want to avoid white bleached foods like bleached flour, white rice, white granulated sugar and white eggs.

Vitamins and Minerals

Vitamin C

Getting at least 600mg daily of whole complex vitamin C, not ascorbic acid derived from GMO-corn, found in powdered or frozen purees of Camu-camu, Acerola cherry, and Kakadu is essential for health and the immune system. The immune system is your first line of defense against cancer.

Vitamin C, or ascorbic acid, is a water-soluble vitamin well known for its role in supporting a healthy immune system. Because your body cannot make vitamin C, it must come from the foods you eat every day. Research shows vitamin C is essential for the growth and repair of tissue all over the body.

According to the National Cancer Institute (NCI), vitamin C may protect against cancer of the oral cavity, stomach, and esophagus and may also reduce the risk of developing cancers of the rectum, pancreas, and cervix. Also known as ascorbic acid, vitamin C may provide protection against breast and lung cancer.

Vitamin D

Its popular knowledge that vitamin D as the vitamin important for bone health and for preventing rickets in children, the major source of vitamin D is ultraviolet light from the sun. By definition vitamin D is actually a hormone. Once you create vitamin D in your skin, or ingest it from your diet, it goes to your liver, where it's converted to 25-hydroxy- vitamin D known as calcidiol and then transported to the kidneys to be converted to it's active form, 1,25-dihydroxy-vitamind D, also known as calcitriol.

Vitamin D is very important in helping you use the calcium in your diet by increasing intestinal calcium absorption, and to help mineralize the skeleton to have healthy bones. But, we are now also recognizing that many cells in the body, separate from the kidneys, can activate vitamin D and there is mounting evidence that that function of vitamin D is to help regulate cellular growth. There are several studies that have related higher blood levels of 25-hydroxyvitamin D and reduced-risk of many deadly cancers including colon, breast, and prostate cancer to name a few.

According to vitamin D scholar dr. Holick taking 4000-5000 IUs daily of D3 is optimal. But taking 2000-3000 IU of vitamin D3 a day from dietary sources, sensible sun exposure and supplements is also adequate. Vitamin K2 can inhibit the progression of liver cancer. K2 should be taken along with Vitamin D, 100mg per 10,000 IU's of vitamin d, to keep the calcium within the bones. However, the mechanism of VK2 in inhibiting HCC cell proliferation is not clear.

If you take note of the graph below, you can see that maintaining a 25-hydroxy-vitamin D serum blood level between 40-60 ng/ml prevent a majority of diseases including many cancers.

Magnesium

Magnesium is a critical mineral that is involved in well over 600 enzymatic functions, including those important for brain, heart, and skeletal muscle functions. Because of a deficiency of magnesium in commercial farms soils about 60% of Americans are deficient in magnesium, including up to 60% of patients who are critically ill.

In regard to cancer, magnesium intake has been associated with the reduced incidences of some cancers and has been studied as a protective agent against chemotherapy-induced nephrotoxicity.

Colorectal Cancer

Several studies have demonstrated an association between high magnesium intake and reduced risk of colorectal cancer (CRC).

An analysis of the prospective, Swedish Mammography Cohort, evaluated 61,433 women aged 40 to 75 without a history of cancer for a mean follow-up of 14.8 years. The group with the highest intake of magnesium was associated with a significantly lower risk of CRC compared with the group taking the lowest amount of magnesium. This benefit was observed for both colon and rectal cancers.

A case-control study evaluated 2204 subjects from the Tennessee Colorectal Polyp Study, which demonstrated that increasing total magnesium intake was significantly associated with decreasing risk of CRC (highest tertile odds

ratio [OR], 0.54; 95% CI, 0.36-0.82; $P < .01$).3
The highest tertile of dietary magnesium intake
(>298 mg/day) was significantly associated with
reduced risk of CRC in an age-adjusted model
(OR, 0.75; 95% CI, 0.60-0.95; $P = .02$).

A study of 140,601 postmenopausal women from
the Women's Health Initiative with an mean
follow-up of 13 years demonstrated a significant
reduction in CRC risk with the highest intake of
total magnesium intake compared with the lowest
intake of magnesium intake.

Pancreatic Cancer

A study of 66,806 subjects aged 50 to 76 at
baseline from the Vitamins and Lifestyle cohort
evaluated magnesium intake and the incidence of
pancreatic cancer during a mean follow-up of 6.8
years. Six Subjects with magnesium intake below
the recommended dietary allowance were more
likely to develop pancreatic cancer, particularly in
those whose intake was less than 75% of the
recommended dietary allowance. In this study, a
100 mg/day decrease in magnesium intake
resulted in a 24% increase in risk of pancreatic
cancer.

Nephrotoxicity

Several studies have demonstrated that magnesium administered during chemotherapy treatment has a protective effect against nephrotoxicity.

A double-blind, placebo-controlled phase 2 study randomly assigned 40 patients with epithelial ovarian cancer to receive magnesium sulphate (5 g) before each course of chemotherapy (paclitaxel plus cisplatin) with magnesium subcarbonate (500 mg 3 times per day) administered during treatment intervals. Magnesium supplementation was effective in increasing serum magnesium levels, and resulted in a significantly lower decrease in glomerular filtration rate (GFR) compared with placebo as indicated by serum creatinine, Cockroft-Gault , and Modification Diet of Renal Disease.

A study of 85 patients with lung cancer receiving cisplatin-based chemotherapy received high or low volume hydration with magnesium or high volume hydration without magnesium. The group that did not receive magnesium demonstrated a significant increase in serum creatinine and significant decrease in creatinine clearance compared with baseline. There was no difference in serum creatinine or creatinine clearance compared with baseline for patients who received high volume hydration with magnesium, and a trend toward increased serum creatinine and decreased creatinine clearance in the group that receive low volume hydration with magnesium.

Anti-oxidants

Antioxidants are substances that inhibit the oxidation process and act as protective agents. They protect the body from the damaging effects of free radicals (by-products of the body's normal chemical processes). Free radicals attack healthy cells, which changes their DNA, allowing tumors to grow.

Beta carotene

Beta carotene, also known as provitamin A, may help decrease the risk of developing cancer. According to the American Cancer Society, this nutrient may prevent certain cancers by enhancing the white blood cells in your immune system. White blood cells work to block cell-damaging free radicals.

Good sources of beta carotene are dark green leafy and yellow-orange fruits and vegetables. In the body, beta carotene is converted to vitamin A. Eating foods rich in beta carotene is recommended to possibly decrease the risk of developing stomach, lung, prostate, breast, and head and neck cancer.

However, more research is needed before a definite
recommendation on beta carotene consumption can be made. Overdosing on beta carotene is not recommended. Large doses can cause the skin to turn a yellow-orange color, a condition called carotenosis. High intakes of beta carotene in supplement form may actually cause lung cancer in people at risk, such as smokers.

While there is a recommended dietary allowance for vitamin A, there is not one for beta carotene. Examples of some foods high in beta carotene include the following:

Carrots
Squash
Collards
Spinach
Sweet potatoes

Vitamin E

Vitamin E is essential for our bodies to work properly. Vitamin E helps to build normal and red blood cells, as well as working as an antioxidant. Research is finding evidence that vitamin E may protect against prostate and colorectal cancer. The recommended dietary allowance for vitamin E is 15 milligrams per day. The adult upper limit for vitamin E is 1,000 milligrams per day. Good sources of vitamin E (and the amount each serving contains) include the following:

- 1 tablespoon sunflower oil - 6.9 mg
- 1 ounce sunflower seeds - 14 mg
- 1 ounce almonds - 7.4 mg
- 1 ounce hazelnuts - 4.3 mg
- 1 ounce peanuts - 2.1 mg
- 3/4 cup bran cereal - 5.1 mg
- 1 slice whole wheat bread - .23 mg
- 1 ounce wheat germ - 5.1 mg

Chapter 3

Natural Substances to Remove Cancer

Lemons

Well chugging down lemon water is not really going to significantly fight cancer, though it will rid your Rheumatoid arthritis, but that's another story for another day. What we're really interested in is what's concentrated in the skin of lemons...D-limonene.

D-Limonene is a common terpene in nature. It's not just in lemon skins, it's also present in several citrus skins such as orange, lemon, mandarin, lime, and grapefruit. The US National Library of Medicine has animal studies where D-Limonene has shown amazing ability to neutralize, inhibit or cause apoptosis to a wide variety of cancers. Preliminary studies in humans are also showing promising results.

There are two ways to get D-Limonene, one you can buy an extract like Jarrows D-Limonene, or you can juice organic Lemon peels or the whole lemon daily. It's important if you take the Lemon skin route that the lemons are organic:

1. If lemons are grown with pesticide use, the lemon tree stops producing D-Limonene.

2. D-Limonene is produced by the tree as an anti-fungal.
3. You don't want to hamper your liver with more poisonous pesticides if you are fighting cancer.

Suggested Dosage:

Using a blender and juice 1 whole organic lemon once or twice daily in two cups of juice such as orange juice. Drink immediately or throughout the day.

Powdered Black Seeds & Black Seed Oil(nigella sativa)

Powdered black seeds is one of the most incredible natural substances I've discovered. Unfortunately it's also one of the most ignored plants in nature by the pharmaceutical industry due to its "heal all" capabilities. There are thousands of research articles on PubMed elucidating its health giving properties, especially relating to cancer. *Nigella sativa* has been used as traditional medicine for centuries. The crude oil and the thymoquinone extracted from its seeds and oil are effective against many diseases like cancer, cardiovascular complications, diabetes, asthma, and kidney disease etc. Thymoquinone, the main bioactive component of Nigella sativa, has been found to exhibit anticancer effects in numerous preclinical studies. Due to its multitargeting nature, thymoquinone interferes in a wide range of tumorigenic processes and counteracts carcinogenesis, malignant growth, invasion, migration, and angiogenesis. Moreover, thymoquinone can specifically sensitize tumor cells toward conventional cancer treatments (e.g., radiotherapy, chemotherapy, and immunotherapy) and simultaneously minimize therapy-associated toxic effects in normal cells.

Black seed oil has been shown to be effective against cancer in blood system, lung, kidney, liver, prostate, breast, cervix, skin with much safety. *The molecular mechanisms behind its anticancer role is still not clearly understood,* however, some studies showed that thymoquinone has an antioxidant role and improves body's defense system, induces apoptosis of cancer cells and controls Akt pathway.

In the Pubmed article,"Anticancer Activities of Nigella Sativa (Black Cumin)" it states the many cancers Black seed oil is effective against -

Thymoquinone = TQ

Blood Cancer

El-Mahdy et al. (2005) reported that TQ exhibits anti-proliferative effect in human myeloblastic leukemia HL-60 cells. Derivatives of TQ bearing terpene-terminated 6-alkyl residues were tested in HL-60 cells and 518A2 melanoma by Effenberger et al. (2010). They found the derivatives induce apoptosis associated with DNA laddering, a decrease in mitochondrial membrane potential and a slight increase in reactive oxygen species. Swamy and Huat (2003) observed that α-hederin also induced death of murine leukemia P388 cells by a dose- and time-dependent increase in apoptosis.

Breast Cancer

Aqueous and alcohol extracts of *N. sativa* were found to be effective *in vitro* in inactivating MCF-7 breast cancer cells (Farah and Begum, 2003). *N. sativa*, in combination with melatonin and retinoic acid reduced the carcinogenic effects of DMBA (7, 12-di-methylbenz(a)anthracene) in mammary carcinoma of rats (El-Aziz et al., 2005). Terpene-terminated 6-alkyl residues of TQ were tested in MCF-7/Topo breast carcinoma by

Effenberger et al. (2010). They found the derivatives inducing cell death by apoptosis.

Colon Cancer

Gali-Muhtasib et al. (2004) suggested that TQ is anti-neoplastic and pro-apoptotic against colon cancer cell line HCT116. Salim and Fukushima (2003) demonstrated that the volatile oil of *N. sativa* has the ability to inhibit colon carcinogenesis of rats in the post-initiation stage, with no evident adverse side effects. Norwood et al. (2006) suggested TQ as chemotherapeutic agent on SW-626 colon cancer cells, in potency, which is similar to 5-flurouracil in action. However, on HT-29 (colon adenocarcinoma) cell, no effect of TQ was found (Rooney and Ryan, 2005).

Pancreatic Cancer

Chehl et al. (2009) showed that TQ, the major constituent of *N. sativa* oil extract, induced apoptosis and inhibited proliferation in PDA (pancreatic ductal adenocarcinoma) cells. They also suggested TQ as a novel inhibitor of pro-inflammatory pathways, which provides a promising strategy that combines anti-inflammatory and proapoptotic modes of action. TQ also can abrogate gemcitabine- or oxaliplatin-induced activation of NF-kappa B, resulting in the chemosensitization of pancreatic tumors to conventional therapeutics (Banerjee et al., 2009). The high molecular weight glycoprotein mucin 4 (MUC4) is aberrantly expressed in pancreatic cancer and contributes to the regulation of differentiation, proliferation, metastasis, and the chemoresistance of pancreatic cancer cells. Torres et al. (2010) evaluated the down-regulatory effect of TQ on MUC4 in pancreatic cancer cells. But in a study, Rooney and Ryan (2005) did not find any preventive role of TQ on MIA PaCa-2 (pancreas carcinoma) cells.

Hepatic Cancer

The cytotoxic activity of *N. sativa* seed was tested on the human hepatoma HepG2 cell line by Thabrew et al. (2005), and 88% inhibitory effect on HepG2 was found after 24-hr incubation with different concentrations (0–50 mg/ml) of the *N. sativa* extract. Nagi and Almakki (2009) reported that oral administration of TQ is effective in increasing the activities of quinone reductase and glutathione transferase and makes TQ a promising prophylactic agent against chemical carcinogenesis and toxicity in hepatic cancer.

Lung Cancer

Swamy and Huat (2003) mentioned the antitumor activity of α-hederin from *N. sativa* against LL/2 (Lewis Lung carcinoma) in BDF1 mice. Also, Mabrouk et al. (2002) showed that supplementation of diet with honey and *N. sativa* has a protective effect against MNU (methylnitrosourea)-induced oxidative stress, inflammatory response and carcinogenesis in lung, skin and colon.

Skin Cancer

Topical application of *N. sativa* extract inhibited two-stage initiation/promotion [dimethylbenz[a]anthracene (DMBA)/croton oil] skin carcinogenesis in mice. Again, intraperitoneal administration of *N. sativa* (100 mg/kg body wt) 30 days after subcutaneous administration of MCA (20-methylcholanthrene) restricted soft tissue sarcomas to 33.3% compared with 100% in MCA-treated controls (Salomi et al., 1991).

Fibrosarcoma

TQ from *N. sativa* was administrated (0.01% in drinking water) one week before and after MCA treatment significantly inhibited the tumor incidence (fibrosarcoma) and tumor burden by 43% and 34%, respectively, compared with the results in the group receiving MCA alone. Moreover, TQ delayed the onset of MCA-induced fibrosarcoma tumors. Also *in vitro* studies showed that TQ inhibited the survival of fibrosarcoma cells with IC50 of 15 mM (Badary and Gamal, 2001). Oil of *N. sativa* also decreased the fibrinolytic potential of the human fibrosarcoma cell line (HT1080) *in vitro* (Awad, 2005).

Renal Cancer

Khan and Sultana (2005) reported the chemo-preventive effect of *N. sativa* against ferric nitrilotriacetate (Fe-NTA)-induced renal oxidative stress, hyper-proliferative response and renal carcinogenesis. Treatment of rats orally with *N. sativa* (50 100 mg/kg body wt) resulted in significant decrease in H_2O_2 generation, DNA synthesis and incidence of tumors.

Prostate Cancer

TQ, from *N. sativa,* inhibited DNA synthesis, proliferation, and viability of cancerous (LNCaP, C4-B, DU145, and PC-3) but not non-cancerous (BPH-1) prostate epithelial cells by down-regulating AR (androgen receptor) and E2F-1 (a transcription factor) (Kaseb et al., 2007). In this study, they suggested TQ as effective in treating hormone-sensitive as well as hormone-refractory prostate cancer. Yi et al. (2008) found that TQ blocked angiogenesis *in vitro* and *in vivo,* prevented tumor angiogenesis in a xenograft human prostate cancer (PC3) model in mouse, and inhibited human prostate tumor growth at low dosage with almost no chemotoxic side effects. Furthermore, they observed that endothelial cells were more sensitive to TQ-induced cell apoptosis, cell proliferation, and migration inhibition compared with PC3 cancer cells. TQ also inhibited vascular endothelial growth factor-induced extracellular signal-regulated kinase activation but showed no inhibitory effects on vascular endothelial growth factor receptor 2 activation.

Cervical Cancer

Shafi et al. (2009) reported that methanol, n-Hexane and chloroform extracts of *N. sativa* effectively killed HeLa (human epithelial cervical cancer) cells by inducing apoptosis. Effenberger et al. (2010) tested terpene-terminated 6-alkyl residues of TQ on multidrug-resistant KB-V1/Vb1 cervical carcinoma and found the derivatives inducing cell death by apoptosis.

Suggested Dosage

I have observed that ingesting two teaspoons to one tablespoon of organic cold-pressed black seed oil twice daily on an empty stomach in a half cup of juice to be effective in eradicating cancer from the body. If you choose to use the organic powdered black seeds which is a more wholistic approach, one to two teaspoons of powdered black seeds mixed in a ½ cup of juice to be very effective. Organic Powdered Black Seeds can be purchased on my website Nothingsincurable.com.

Diatomaceous Earth

I'm not exactly sure how diatomaceous earth removes cancer, but I've encountered many anedoctal testimonies of its efficacy in removing skin and colon cancer.

It's possible by removing all the heavy metals, candida and parasites in the intestines and colon has an indirect on cancer proliferation.

Diatomaceous earth is made from the fossilized remains of microscopic aquatic organisms called diatoms. Their skeletons are predominantly composed of a natural substance called silica. Over millions of years diatoms accumulated in the sediment of rivers, streams, lakes, and oceans. Silica is very common in nature and makes up 26% of the earth's crust by weight. Various forms of silica include sand, emerald, quartz, feldspar, mica, clay, asbestos, and glass. Silicon, a component of silica, does not exist naturally in its pure form. It reacts with oxygen and water to form silicon dioxide, silicon dioxide has two naturally occurring forms: **crystalline** and **amorphous**. Food grade freshwater diatomaceous earth is made of amorphous silicon dioxide.

What is the health benefit of ingesting Diatomaceous Earth?

Essentially diatomaceous earth is like liquid plumber. Because of its abrasiveness, absorption properties, and negative charge, it kills internal parasites, intestinal worms, including candida by dehydration and cutting them up, while also removing heavy metals, and other dangerous microorganisms(viruses and bacteria). By cleaning out your intestines, it allows your intestines to better be able to absorb nutrients.

Is inhaling Diatomaceous Earth dangerous?

Many people are claiming on the internet that breathing in diatomaceous earth is dangerous, let me clear up this misinformation. As I previously stated you have **crystalline** and **amorphous** diatomaceous earth. If you inhale amorphous diatomaceous earth, it's rapidly eliminated from the lung tissue. However, crystalline diatomaceous earth is much smaller, and it may accumulate in lung tissue and lymph nodes, this can be dangerous.

Long-term inhalation of the crystalline form is associated with silicosis, chronic bronchitis, and other respiratory problems. The bulk of diatomaceous earth is amorphous, not crystalline. Food grade diatomaceous earth is **amorphous** and not **crystalline**.

Grades of Diatomaceous Earth

The Diatom is what makes diatomaceous earth special. The amorphous diatom shell's shape and hardness are important to how it works. Fossilized diatom shells that are and have maintained their tubular shape are critical to their effectiveness, and they are found in freshwater deposits. Saltwater deposits contain a mixture of diatom types with different shapes, their fossilized shells are fragile and break easily, which renders them ineffective for health purposes.

Freshwater diatomaceous earth's hardness keeps it from dissolving in liquid and its tubular shape and holes along the diatom's wall allow it to absorb moisture. The diatomaceous earth you want should consist of at least 89% (and often more) of Silicon Dioxide plus numerous trace minerals. The highest grade of diatomaceous earth appears almost pure white when dry and appears light tan when wet. The lower grades of diatomaceous earth often contain an excess of a mineral and sediment such as iron or a high percentage of clay giving it a darker color or a reddish tint. You want to avoid the darker diatomaceous earth, as it can cause chronic constipation, as well as not possessing the negative charge which attracts bacteria and viruses in the shell of the diatom to be excreted out of the body.

Health Benefits of Diatomaceous Earth

In its pure natural state, diatomaceous earth is an abundant source of Silica and it contains a number of essential minerals. Silica is the most fundamental part of all cells and organisms, so it has a significant benefit. It is an essential component for making muscles, ligaments, cartilage, digestive tract, skin, hair and nails.

Coincidentally, in this PubMed article" The chemistry of silica and its potential health benefits", states that - "Compelling data suggest that silica is essential for health although no RDI has been established. However, deficiency induces deformities in the skull and peripheral bones, poorly formed joints, reduced contents of cartilage, collagen, and disruption of mineral balance in the femur and vertebrae."

Diatomaceous earth offers an alternative method for detoxing your body, it's cheap, simple, and effective. It doesn't require fasting, and many people have used it with great success. Its naturally absorbent and abrasive nature makes it an ideal internal cleaner. As it passes through your system, it absorbs harmful toxins, and it does this without requiring you to change your diet or lifestyle. Another benefit is to use it as a colon cleanse. It functions to eliminate intestinal viruses, parasites, and toxic residues.

It can be used as a food supplement to improve blood cholesterol, mental clarity and enhance energy. It can also be used as an effective treatment for curing hemorrhoids, insomnia, arthritis, back pain, and more. Besides all this, diatomaceous earth is also widely used in a range of skincare and cosmetic products.

What Is The Herxheimer Reaction

The Herxheimer Reaction is an immune system response to the toxins that are released when large amounts of pathogens are being killed off, and the body does not eliminate the toxins quickly enough. It's simply a reaction that occurs when the body is detoxifying and the released toxins either exacerbate the symptoms being treated or create their own symptoms. The important thing to note is that worsening symptoms are not an indicator of the failure of the treatment; in fact, usually just the opposite, it means it's working.

Some of the symptoms include:

- **Headache**
- **Flu-like symptoms**
- **Itch and rashes**
- **Flushes**

Cleansing instructions

The protocol of taking diatomaceous earth varies from person to person, but typically you want to start with a small amount on an empty stomach, either in the morning or in the evening. When I first started my diatomaceous earth regimen, I started with ½ teaspoon stirred in with orange juice before I went to bed. But some people start with a teaspoon, I wouldn't advise initially taking more than a teaspoon.

The purpose of taking diatomaceous earth at night is the potential of bowel movements during the initial cleansing period.

The daily dosage should be increased by half or a quarter teaspoon every few days until you can ingest one tablespoon daily.

It is very important to drink lots of water, preferably natural alkaline water, not ionized water, I used Evamor. The reason being is diatomaceous earth can be dehydrating, and the water aids the kidneys to flush out the toxins and parasites. Many of the toxins being released into the bloodstream are acidic, and the alkaline water will also neutralize them.

Some people will experience the herx response the first time they ingest diatomaceous earth, some get it a week later or even longer. Sometimes the herx response happens when you're ingesting at least one tablespoon a day. If you still have not experienced the Herx response with one tablespoon a day try two tablespoons, once in the evening and one in the morning. If you still do not experience the herx response, it most likely means your cleansing detox was much lighter, and you are not going to experience it at all.

About a week after the body experiences the herx response, your intestines should now be optimal for nutrient absorption.

Diatomaceous earth can be purchased on my website Nothingsincuble.com

I will make an honorary mention of guinea hen weed, and soursop leaves. Both possess phytochemicals that directly kill cancer cells. But in my opinion neither of them have the anti-cancer efficacy as powdered blacks seeds or lemons rinds.

Chapter 4

Rebuild the body

The fallacy of *ascorbic acid* being labeled as Vitamin C is one of the greatest health impediments to humans in modern times. In reality, ascorbic acid is actually just one component of whole complex vitamin C. Vitamin C operates as a complex of multiple factors of which ascorbic acid is just one, it acts as an antioxidant wrapper for choline, rutin, the enzyme tyrosinase, vitamin K, and bioflavonoids(vitamin P) a powerful family of over 6,000 antioxidants that have a symbiotic working relationship within vitamin C, with each increasing the other's effect. Without these cofactors, vitamin C cannot perform its true health benefits in the body. Whole complex vitamin C is found in varying degrees in a wide variety of fruits and vegetables, but vitamin C is at incredibly high and therapeutic levels in camu-camu, a South American superfood that resembles a grape.

Camu-camu is what you need to rebuild your body, and is second only to kakadu plum in whole complex vitamin C. It has about 2,000 mg per 100 g fruit (spray-dried powder – 10,200 mg) – or almost 34 times of the recommended daily intake! It is also ranked among the top foods in antioxidant value, possessing 52,000 µ mol TE/100g.

Why You Should Beware of Ascorbic Acid: Synthetic Vitamin C

Apparently, an estimated 95% of the world's vitamin C is produced in China. Ascorbic acid is synthesized using a process involving primarily GMO corn and volatile acids.

Whole Vs. Isolated

Most sources equate vitamin C with ascorbic acid, but they're not. Ascorbic acid is an isolate, a fraction, a distillate of naturally whole complex vitamin C. Real vitamin C, whole complex vitamin C is composed of ascorbic acid, rutin, bioflavonoids, vitamin K, choline, and tyrosinase.

In addition, mineral co-factors must be available in proper amounts. If any of these cofactors are missing, there is no true vitamin C activity within the body. When some of them are present, the body will draw on its own stores to make up the difference, so that the whole vitamin may be present. Only then will vitamin activity take place, provided that all other conditions and co-factors are present. Ascorbic acid is described merely as the "antioxidant wrapper" portion of vitamin C; ascorbic acid protects the functional parts of the vitamin from rapid oxidation or breakdown.

Nutritional composition of Camu-Camu

Pioneering work on the high L-ascorbic acid (vitamin C) content of camu-camu fruits was published in 1964. In this report, the authors indicate that camu-camu fruits are among the highest natural sources of vitamin C. These fruits are composed of nutrients such as protein, carbohydrate, lipids, ash, and crude fiber. Additionally, they have essential amino acids (valine, leucine, phenylalanine, etc.), essential fatty acids of the families omega 3 and 6, vitamin C, and vitamins of the B-complex and several essential minerals for human nutrition, such as potassium, phosphorous, sulfate, calcium, magnesium, cobalt, iron, and several others.

Health-promoting phytochemicals of Camu-camu

An ethnopharmacological survey of medicinal plants in the northeastern Amazon region of Peru showed that several botanical parts of camu-camu such as immature and mature fruits, stems, leaves, roots, seeds, and barks are used to prepare remedies in folk medicine to treat numerous diseases such as arthritis, diabetes, hypercholesterolemia, bronchitis, inflammation, asthma, atherosclerosis, cataracts, depression, flu, gingivitis, glaucoma, hepatitis, infertility, migraine, osteoporosis, Parkinson's disease, and malaria. Additionally, camu-camu is used traditionally for the treatment of malaria by indigenous people of South America. All these traditional uses are in concordance with multiple scientific research showing that several botanical parts of camu-camu are a rich source of various health-promoting phytochemicals with proven health beneficial properties. In addition to vitamin C, several secondary metabolites exist such as polyphenols, carotenoids, bioactive phytochemicals, and other chemicals.

Health Benefits of Vitamin C

Vitamin C promotes healthy mitochondria function, helping the synthesis of ATP energy molecules. It stimulates the immune system to produce interferon and to increase the number of natural killer cells. It optimizes phagocytosis and leukocyte migration, putting the immune system in defensive action. It reduces oxidative damage to gene TP53, which is a gene that creates the protein P53 which acts as a tumor/cancer suppressor, which means that it regulates cell division by keeping cells from growing and dividing (proliferating) too fast or in an uncontrolled way. It has an important influence on the body's defense system to modulate the activity of cells such as leukocytes and macrophages. It improves wound healing and reduces the symptoms caused by allergic reactions. It acts in the body as a carrier of oxygen and hydrogen and has antioxidant action against harmful effects of free radicals associated with the development of tumor, cardiovascular and neurological diseases. It participates actively in liver detoxification processes facilitating the elimination of toxins. Vitamin C helps in the conversion of amino acid neurotransmitters; therefore it exerts an antidepressant action.

It participates in the synthesis of steroid hormones essential for healthy aging and is responsible for metabolism and fat oxidation (lipid) form. It's involved in maintaining the integrity of gums, bones, teeth, and blood vessels. It can effectively combat the flu, allergies, asthma, bronchitis, and other respiratory problems.

In this research article on PubMed " Synthetic or Food-Derived Vitamin C—Are They Equally Bioavailable?", they concluded that there was an immensely increased health benefit in ingesting whole complex vitamin c found in foods in comparison to synthetic ascorbic acid.

Although synthetic and food-derived vitamin C appear to be equally bioavailable in humans, ingesting vitamin C as part of a whole food is considered preferable because of the concomitant consumption of numerous other macro- and micronutrients and phytochemicals, which will confer additional health benefits. Numerous epidemiological studies have indicated that higher intakes of fruit and vegetables are associated with decreased incidence of stroke [100], coronary heart disease [101], and cancers at various sites [102,103]. Vitamin C status is one of the best markers for fruit and vegetable intake [104], and food-derived vitamin C is associated with decreased incidence of numerous chronic diseases [1],

In this Pubmed article,"Tropical fruit camu-camu (Myrciaria dubia) has anti-oxidative and anti-inflammatory properties", they compare the anti-oxidative and anti-inflammatory properties of camu- camu and ascorbic acid with 20 male smokers -

"Methods*: To assess the anti-oxidative and anti-inflammatory properties of camu-camu in humans, 20 male smoking volunteers, considered to have an accelerated oxidative stress state, were recruited and randomly assigned to take daily 70 ml of 100% camu-camu juice, corresponding to 1050 mg of vitamin C (camu-camu group; n=10) or 1050 mg of vitamin C tablets (vitamin C group; n=10) for 7 days.*

Results*: After 7 days, oxidative stress markers such as the levels of urinary 8-hydroxy-deoxyguanosine (P<0.05) and total reactive oxygen species (P<0.01) and inflammatory markers such as serum levels of high sensitivity C reactive protein (P<0.05), interleukin (IL)-6 (P<0.05), and IL-8 (P<0.01) decreased significantly in the camu-camu group,* *while there was no change in the vitamin C group.*

Conclusions*: Our results suggest that camu-camu juice may have powerful anti-oxidative and anti-inflammatory properties, compared to vitamin C tablets containing equivalent vitamin C content. These effects may be due to the existence of unknown anti-oxidant substances besides vitamin C or unknown substances modulating in vivo vitamin C kinetics in camu-camu."*

The article concludes that ingesting the "equivalent" amount of ascorbic acid, which is classified as vitamin C, had no effect on the smokers. But the Camu-camu which possessed real whole complex vitamin C possessed powerful anti-oxidative and anti-inflammatory properties.

Instructions

Camu-camu doesn't dissolve in liquids, and it's also very tart in light of its high vitamin C content. I prefer to mix 1 teaspoon twice a day in a half cup orange juice, once in the morning before I eat or drink anything, and once before I go to bed.

I have found that Camu powder with less than 600mg of vitamin c per teaspoon to be ineffective.

I personally use it every day, and since I've been using it, and everyone else that I coerced into taking it daily, none of us has gotten sick from anything bacterial or viral infection.

I theorize that if we have the correct amount of real whole complex vitamin C constantly flowing in our veins, people would not get sick from anything.

I believe this is also why the Pharmaceutical industry pushes synthetic ascorbic acid over real whole complex vitamin C on the masses.

If you think about it, if you don't constantly have sick people. How will the pharmaceutical corporations, "doctors", and specialized medical clinics stay in business?

Organic raw powdered camu-camu can be purchased on my website.

Nothingsincurable.com.

Endnotes

Cancer is not terrifying. I have seen people in hospice and stage 4 cancer use the methods described above and become cancer free within a couple of months. Everything we need is in nature. We only need to open our eyes and reclaim our lost plant and mineral kingdom knowledge for us to live fulfilling and healthy lives.

About the Author

I am a passionate alternative health researcher and blogger.I also maintain a holistic health website @Nothingsincurable.com.

I have absolutely no formal education in alternative health or nutrition. Meaning I haven't been conditioned in thought or belief. Everything I know I learned on my own through research and self-experimentation. But I did attend University, Florida International University, and I received a Liberal Arts Degree, studying primarily history & anthropology. My journey in Alternative health began years ago with my own ailments, and my desire to find alternatives to the nightmare of harmful & addictive pharmaceutical drugs, and the never ending trail of health insurance bills and co-payments.

What I discovered I passed on to my friends and relatives. So that they too could naturally heal from their diseases and chronic ailments. Eventually, I developed a burning desire to share my knowledge with the world, and I started my health blog.

Bibliography:

https://www.ncbi.nlm.nih.gov/pmc/articles/PMC4702494/

https://www.sciencedirect.com/science/article/pii/S0304389422009578?via%3Dihub

https://www.foodpackagingforum.org/news/scientists-identify-most-harmful-food-contact-chemicals

https://ehjournal.biomedcentral.com/articles/10.1186/s12940-019-0488-0#:~:text=Of%20the%2025%20most%20commonly,the%20EU%2C%20China%20and%20Brazil.

https://www.safecosmetics.org/chemicals/known-carcinogens/

https://www.sciencedirect.com/science/article/abs/pii/S1383574218300887

https://www.cnn.com/2019/02/14/health/us-glyphosate-cancer-study-scli-intl/index.html

https://www.ncbi.nlm.nih.gov/pmc/articles/PMC2990475/#:~:text=Indeed%2C%20cancer%20initiation%20and%20progression,and%20cell%20proliferation%20%5B11%5D.

The Vitamin D Solution

https://www.ncbi.nlm.nih.gov/pmc/articles/PMC2715207/

https://www.ncbi.nlm.nih.gov/books/NBK507261
/

https://stanfordhealthcare.org/medical-clinics/can
cer-nutrition-services/reducing-cancer-risk/antiox
idants.html

https://www.frontiersin.org/articles/10.3389/fonc.
2021.757603/full#:~:text=Vitamin%20K2%20(V
K2)%2C%20a,cell%20proliferation%20is%20not
%20clear.

Made in the USA
Middletown, DE
01 June 2024

55158072R00046